BEFORE AFTER
THE ACCIDENTAL
DIETITIAN

FROM MENTAL ILLNESS
TO HEALTHY BODY AND MIND
LIFE CHANGING STORY
WEIGHT LOSS DIET PLANS

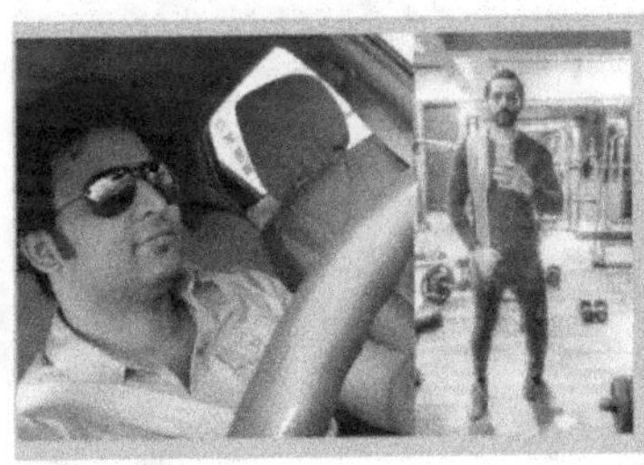

KHAWAR KHAN

FAMOUS FITNESS YOUTUBER,
INFLUENCER,
TELEVISION PRODUCER AND
A WEIGHT MANAGEMENT
EXPERT

THE ACCIDENTAL DIETITIAN

ISBN: 9798596677805:

DEDICATION

I dedicate this book to every person who is ready and willing to be the better version of himself or herself in all walks of life, not just body-wise.

CONTENTS

ACKNOWLEDGMENTS

I thank everyone who looked down upon me and disregarded my talent as they motivated me to have the courage to be a successful and happy person. Also, I thank my Mother and Wife for always believing in me.

CHAPTER 1 "WHO I'M"

I Don't Know how to label this book an autobiography or a weight loss guide book, but one thing for sure is clear that whoever will read this book will change his/her life and learn how to fight for themselves no matter what.

Readers, this is Khawar Khan, Author of this book, a severe illness survivor (I will share in Chapter 3), and a successful Fitness Youtuber with 160k Subscribers together with hundreds of weight loss videos and diet plans.

A calm soul, changing many lives from sad to happy, from stressed to calm, and from obese to fit.

Naming this book "The Accidental Dietitian" was truly an Accidental thing that you will understand more clearly by reading Chapter 2 and more.

CHAPTER 2 "WHO I WAS"

When I talk about my present, I label myself to be a calm and composed soul.

But I was not the same in my past. When I completed my undergraduate studied in 2008, I started my first job in the media industry, where I loved what I did. I began my fitness journey as well, where I went to the gym, built muscles, gained a healthier lifestyle, and became fit.

I was always very sharp, a go-getter, eager for success, and also aggressive and overthinker.

In the first few years of my Media Jobs, my work and performance were exceptionally great, which led me to many appreciation certificates from Leading Television Network "ARY DIGITAL NETWORK," multiple promotions and increments, life was all set.

I produced Pakistan's Top-rated Morning Show, traveling to many countries, drawing a good monthly salary, and enjoying a dream life big car at the young age of 23.

But at the same time, I was not doing great health-wise

as I was not taking care of my food choices and sleep timing. I used to wake up at 6:30 in the morning, having slept at 2:00 or 3:00 am in the morning, getting only a few hours of sleep.

I never knew these things would take me to a place that

I never knew these things would take me to a place that I never expected without being aware of living with an illness (i will explain in chapter 3) from an early age.

As time passes, I gained a lot of weight from a healthy 72 Kg on 5 Feet 10 inches height gained to 90 Kg.

But without any fear of weight gain, I was working day and night, and one secret I was in a not normal relationship with a lady.

Besides my career and job, I invested and wasted most of my time in this relationship (Long Irrelevant detail, but the reasons we're growing stress, anxiety, and anger).

As you all know, stress can lead you to serious weight gain.

Ups and downs are always part of life as time passes, I left my dream job and broke up with my lady. Switched job again left the job and made my life more uncertain health-wise and career-wise.

One day early in the morning, I felt severe pain in my stomach; it was so much that I had to visit the hospital. They kept me there for a few hours, got my several tests done, and named my pain anxiety and gasses. But the accidental ultrasound finding was that I have fatty liver; by the way, it's not the same illness that I will explain in Chapter 3.

Non-Alcoholic Fatty liver means that you have extra fat in your liver, and the liver is unable to process it and break it.

In present life approx. 25% of the world population suffers from the fatty liver due to an unhealthy diet and lifestyle.

But in some cases, it can lead to NASH and then liver cirrhosis or liver scarring, which can be life-threatening. Most of the 25% of the world population either don't know about their fatty liver or take it as a regular thing and don't google much. But unfortunately, I did, which boosted my anxiety and fear of dying. At that time, I had a lot of fat in my belly area. My doctor advised me to adopt a healthy lifestyle, daily walks, and a healthy diet, but I did not know something bigger would appear soon, which is already there since my childhood, which will take me far away from this liver stress.

CHAPTER 3
"MY ILLNESS AND WEIGHT GAIN"

Let me start it from childhood; we are four siblings, and everyone used to say that I was the best student who always got good grades among the four of us.

When I was ten years old, my parents decided to shift home from Karachi, Pakistan, to another.

 But my school was near the old house, also my maternal grandmother's house.

So, my parents and I decided that I will live at my grandmother's house till the end of the education year, they all moved to the new house, and I moved to my grandmother's.

I was an outstanding student in the sixth standard, but a new habit was developing in me, growing day by day. It was about the obsession with hygiene and germs.

Without knowing its details, I started doing every day activities differently, like washing hands, often demanding a separate food plate, glass, and spoon.

None of my family members or grandmother's family

had any idea that it's a mental illness or that it could be treated or managed.

So, I was suffering from a mental illness called OCD – obsessive-compulsive disorder without knowing anything about it.

To explain this in easier words, I can say that thoughts come into your mind it becomes your obsession, and fulfilling it becomes a compulsion in your mind.

Initially, Symptoms were very little, just separate food Plates, Mug, Spoon. But as I grew, it grew with time, for instance, washing hands after shaking hands with anyone and taking a bath if the smallest droplet from anyone's mouth comes on my cloth during a conversation.

But taking it all as usual as a super hygienic person, I was living my life normally.

In Pakistan, many street food hygiene is terrible, so whenever I used to have any tasty street food, I never looked at the cook because they always do unhygienic stuff like scratching their backs while making burgers. A regular guy would also mind such behavior, but people here use to make fun that it's normal, so one doesn't overthink as I was always confused about hygiene issues.

In my twenties, I had the idea that it can be OCD as I

used to read articles related to it, but I never visited a doctor or psychiatrist for it. As the time passed and I shared in chapter two after leaving one of my highest paid jobs in 2015. I developed anxiety, fear of travel, fear of death, fear of illnesses, hypochondria, depression, and whatnot. Well, these all are in the package of OCD.

I Visited my Gasto-endocrinologist for my continuous stomach disturbance and pain due to IBS irritable bowel syndrome. This common disorder affects the large intestines making an individual always feel cramps, pain, gas, bloating, constipation, or diarrhea. The doctor suggested that I have an extreme anxiety level where I explained to him about my fear of death that I always feel and read about terminal diseases online frequently. I also read about medicines on google and their side effects, which further fuel the anxiety; he suggested me to visit a psychiatrist as I portrayed symptoms of a hypochondriac (fear of illness). Also, he suggested Psyllium Husk (Ispaghol Husk), which is a very high source of the soluble and insoluble fibers of IBS symptoms.

In depression and stress, individuals mostly gain more weight, but some lose weight. I was 90k at that time, with visible belly fat accumulating. But fortunately, this illness and depression worked in my favor. I began to lose weight; maybe I was eating less, thinking much, and taking Ispaghol Husk Daily.

I lost some weight, but that became one more thought of worry that I might have some significant disease due to which I am losing so much weight.

I was still making good money facing all these health problems. I never went to a psychiatrist and started living with these fears, often unnecessary medical tests and visiting doctors due to anxiety and fears from Blood tests to ECG to other tests. And I was not happy as all were normal, but I used to feel different pains.

In 2016 I made more money than ever from freelancing, directing ads, and other media stuff. I took my family, my mother, sister, and both grandparents to Umrah. It's the Holy worship of Muslims in which we visit the holy cities of Makkah and Madina in Saudi Arabia.

There, I prayed for myself. I came back, got married, and started a new job in 2017. After that, I started offering Namaz (Prayer) regularly. It's like a meditation that minimized many of my symptoms, but it was there inside me. I worked usually for one year, and in 2017 December, Allah blessed me with a baby girl. My life was happy and better now; however, I didn't know that the most prominent phase of this OCD is coming forward.

As I used to work for TV, Produced Morning Shows for years and years. I have good terms with many doctors, experts, and mind scientists. To make my life better, I thought of going to a psychologist at the suggestion of a dear brother Dr. Muhammad Imranho. He owns Transformation Centre helping people with mental illness and disorders and changing lives. He suggested that I visit a psychologist in his center to discuss my life and symptoms one day to share these fears with him during the commercial break of my morning show where he was a guest in the show.

I visited the psychologist and took some sessions. Felt better and left due to my job and ever working commitments, brought about by a change in management in May 2018. The TV Channel I was working for shut down the department, and I lost my job.

After a week of it from nowhere, my OCD came back much more potent and destructing. I became a house prisoner and developed an extreme fear of illness and intrusive thoughts. At that time, I had no wish to live life whatever disease I hear or see on tv or the internet. I start feeling the symptoms at that time; my life became miserable when I heard about some people who died from the Bacteria Amoeba Naegleria fowleri or brain-eating amoeba, a germ that enters your brain from the nasal cavity and eats your brain tissues. 99% of people cannot survive from it.

Imagine we Muslims take water in our nose five times a performing ablution before prayer. After every absolution, I used to think that bacteria have found a way into my nose, and I will die. I use to rub my nose from inside out of the paranoia, and it would start bleeding. Even though in the past few years, few cases reported in my city. I used to read this news like a regular guy, but when the thought and fear of this bacteria stuck in my brain in May 2018, it made my life miserable.

I decided to revisit the psychologist. I went to see her, where she suggested some breathing exercises and other stuff; she also suggested I visit a psychiatrist for some medical support. Initially, I was reluctant about medicines, but Dr. Muhammad Imran made me understand that if there is a deficiency of a chemical in the brain, only that chemical would balance it and give you power and support to overcome these intrusive thoughts. In all that time, one of my worst fear was who would deal with and nurture my daughter and who would take care of my family if something goes wrong with me. The best thing in this whole scenario was that I was not ready to give up and to give these thoughts power to make me do something wrong.

I fought by taking sessions and medicines. The reason for telling you all this is related to weight loss, fitness, and a better version of you. Because the only confirmed defeat is when you accept it, and I never wanted to lose, nor will I ever. I fought, and if required in the future, I will fight everything to be the best of me.

CHAPTER 4
"LIFE CHANGING LESSONS "

During my sessions with the psychologist, she felt that I am too much occupied by my fears and anxiety that I don't even spend time with my six-month-old princess and wife.

Her few words changed my life here.

1.   In a conversation, I was telling her that I am fearful that if something goes wrong with me, what would happen to my family, my parents, wife, and daughter. Who would take care of them financially?

She Said

"Tell me one thing, when you were not born, who used to feed your parents? You?"

I said, "No."

She said, "who used to feed your wife and she was single?"

I said, "no of course."

She again said, "who used to feed your parents when

you were very young? You?"

"who has promised every soul for Rizq (food)"

I said, "Allah (God)"

She said, "when Allah (s.w.t.) has taken this responsibility so let him do it and you do what you are here in this world for"

I was quiet but in peace; one of my biggest fears was what would happen to my family if something happens to me, which created many other fears like fear of dying, fear of illness disappearing, and I could feel the change right at that moment.

2.   She asked me, "how old is my daughter."

I said, " she is six months old."

She said, "tell me few things about her how she smiles how she cries."

And at that moment, I was blank because of all the problems that were happening in my life, such as I was spending enough time with my daughter neither taking care of her as much as I wanted.

She added

"Listen Mr. Khawar today your daughter is six months old and you missed many of her beautiful memories.

Which you won't ever be able to see in future so don't miss her beautiful childhood enjoy it otherwise you will only regret it because I know you don't have any illness that would kill you. Nothing will happen to you".

Her words made me realize that once time passed, no one can ever reverse it. I am missing all these beautiful memories in the ifs and buts of my thoughts.

At that moment, I decided to live life. If something is meant to happen, it will happen. If not, why worry.

I started taking medicines and thought to bring change to my life.

And here I am, trying to change other's lives now.

CHAPTER 5
"EVIL EYE AND BLACK MAGIC "

Before I move to the reason for writing this book about my weight loss journey and diet plans, I'd like to add this chapter, and I know many of you reading and inspired by the previous two chapters might disagree with this one or might find me superstitious. But still, I would like to share these experiences of my life.

I am Muslim, and in Islam infect in almost all religions, you will find a bit of agreement upon Black Magic and Evil Eye's reality. Since its existence is mentioned in our Holy Book, we cannot be denied. All I know when everything is going perfect, and suddenly things start going wrong, there can be some negative energy too, whether you name it evil eye, black magic, the negativity of jealous people, or anything else, it's very much there and it exists. In my case, none of my jobs I left got fired due to work performance or my diseases. It all happened so suddenly, either my irrelevant anger, which I got shocked later, why I did so, or people's jealousy and negativity. There are many such stories to tell, but I want to keep this book short and to the point. I want to add that whenever I use to see financial crises,

God Bless my Mother and always keep her with me. She used to pray a lot for me, and her prayers have always taken me out of problems. And one must take all efforts to take the negativity out of like which is in any form and from any solution from meditation to prayer to reading the book of God.

It's very easy to kill Evil Eye and Magic Related things by reciting the Holy Quran's last two chapters in Islam. I did it and took the support of some scholars too.

This chapter's take-home message would be negativity is from negative people, jealous people who cannot bear your success and growth. They will always try to let you down by their words, actions, and other means.

Your goal is to be consistent over your goal and fight.

When I was taking sessions with my psychologist people, some close people see me as if I have gone mad. And some close co-workers started saying in the market to avoid giving him work as he is always sick. So, I am sharing my story in this book with the world because I believe I fought and got control by Allah's grace. But do not tell your weakness to the world; they will always use it against you until you are ready to teach others how to overcome it.

CHAPTER 6
"MY WEIGHT LOSS JOURNEY "

My weight loss journey is not based on a three four-month diet or exercise like you might have read about many transformations and journeys. As I mentioned in earlier chapters, stress and depression worked in my favorites and a lot of study and the right diet, which I will mention in this and further chapters.

Let me give you a quick overview with pictures that when I started my first professional job for a Morning Show back in 2010, I was 22 and I was very fit. I was doing gym trying to build some muscles with significantly less fat on my body.

But within three years of working, waking up at 6 am and sleeping late 2 am or more, not taking food at the right time, and sitting in the office for hours. I gained weight from 73KG approx. to 91 KG.

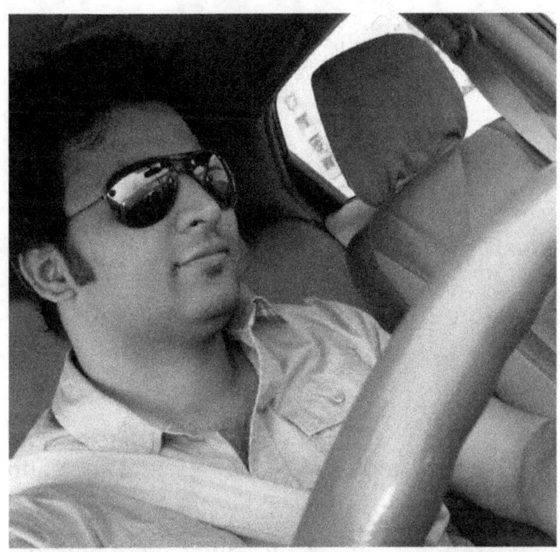

Picture from Sep 2012, I weighed more than 85 KG. At this time, I lost my first job after four years of hard work and health damage and had my first big breakup. So, the first episode of depression and illness already started.

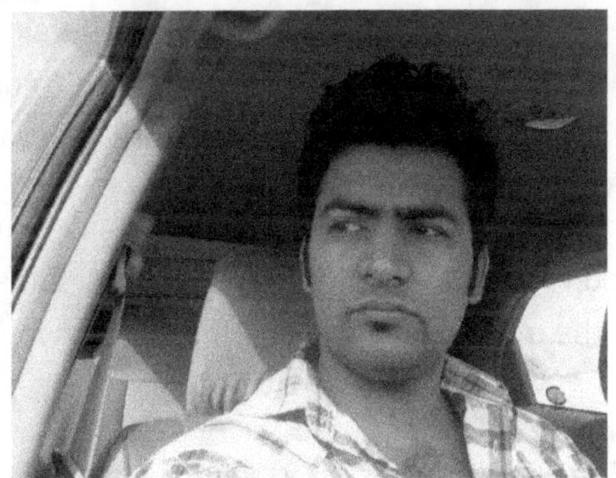

Picture from June 2012, two months before leaving the job.

The reason behind showing these pictures is to have an overview of the weight I gained. One more problem was I could not exercise due to my lower back pain, which was a continuous pain due to my weight and an accident while lifting a deep freezer with my brother to move from one room to another place.

I went to a neuro physician for this pain, and he suggested I not workout and controlled my weight through diet.

I am good with food knowledge, calories, and good and bad fat as I have done morning shows and magazine shows for years and years. Many leading dietitians and doctors of the country used to be guests in the show, also a fitness-related segment in the show.

So, it was the time sitting at home jobless to look for me in the mirror that what I gained and what I lost in 4 years. The quickest answer was my belly J . Literally, when I saw myself in the mirror, the biggest gain apart from traveling many countries, gaining world exposure, and millions of new learnings, was my belly fat.

So, I decided to be the better version of myself and worked on the most listened to and most effective formula.

We say in Pakistan Breakfast like Kings, Lunch like Ministers and Dinner Like Beggars.

So, I started doing better breakfast and less dinner. One formula I read somewhere was, eat in 30 minutes once you wake up and finish your dinner 4 hours before sleep. I started doing that also. And shed some kilos in 2 months along with the stress and tension of not getting another Job. (as I said, stress work in my favor when it comes to weight loss). But in the 3rd month, I got a new job from my previous tv network. I started an even bigger show with an even higher salary and more responsibilities. But this time, along with work, I tried managing my health and weight at least by not eating horrible stuff regularly and eating breakfast. Still, I had no idea about high protein breakfast and macro counts. But I was doing my kind.

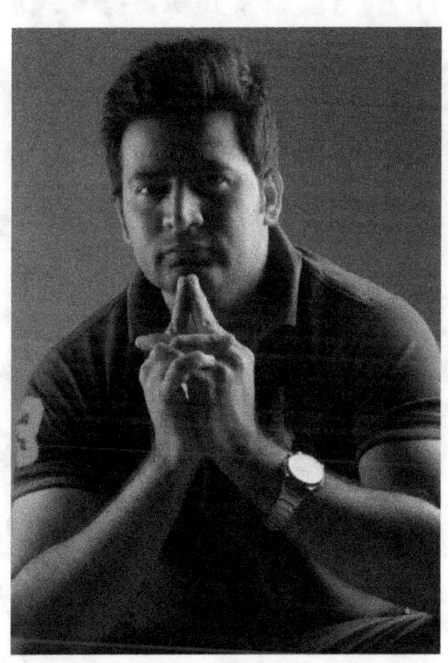

I kept working with a stuck weight near 80 without putting in much effort.

Later in life, the doctor suggested that I have Psyllium (Espagnol husk) to treat my IBS it helped me lose more weight. Along with a high protein breakfast and dinner. As I started looking better leaner and I was losing inches, my interest was much higher reading about weight loss diet recipes, macros, and more. Applying these all things to myself, I got this result.

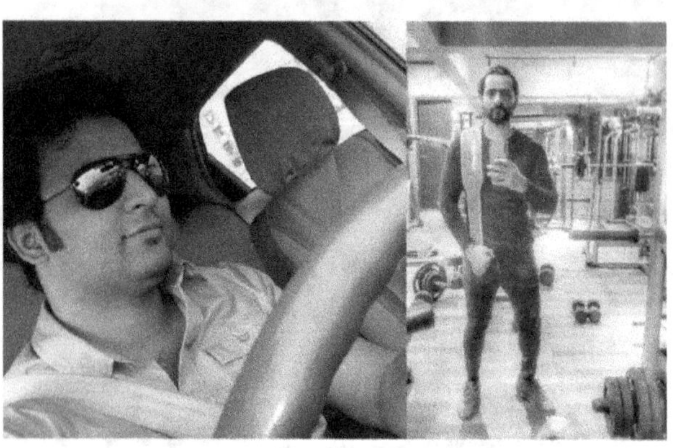

CHAPTER 7
"JOURNEY TO BECOME A VLOGGER"

I had always worked offline, and I had no interest in social media apart from my accounts on Facebook and a blog website I started back in 2014, which is still running with a 730k Facebook page and website. But I had no interest in coming on camera personally for vlogs. But when I got married to the most beautiful person in my life, things changed totally. She is the person who believes in me more than myself or anybody else. I was going through all this pain, anger, and the worst period of OCD when my psychologist asked me to spend time with family and do good for them. I was jobless and had much time to waste or invest. However, I was making money from passive business and managing other YouTube channels.

At that moment, my wife supported me as no lady would. In return, she demanded that she wants to see me as a known and popular personality. She forced me to start vlogs. I was a very shy person though working behind the camera for decades; I had no courage to come in front of the camera. But she was steadfast in her idea that I could do it. And to get me on track, she gave me an idea instead of thinking about fears and OCD. You are good at creating content and already running a blog website and Facebook page. Let's start two-three YouTube channels and Facebook pages. I agreed for her sake. And we made a couple of kids' videos and other videos. Still, her interest was always to bring me in front of the camera, so I made few motivational videos on life relationships and success for Facebook and YouTube, which went well and got a couple of thousand and a few hundred thousand views on Facebook but no significant response on YouTube. People started saying good things about my motivational videos on my Facebook page and sharing their life problems with me. I started feeling good about it.

CHAPTER 8
"THE ACCIDENTAL DIETITIAN "

One day, a lady, I guess, shared about her problem that her marriage is in trouble due to her weight. I do not remember exactly, but I guess I made a video on losing weight due to her comment.

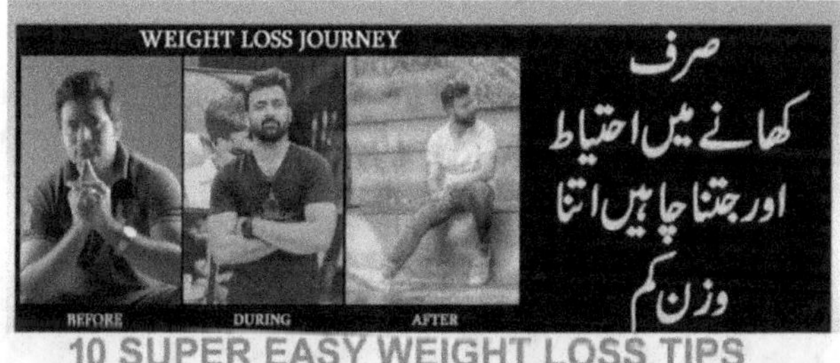

This video got really good YouTube views and helped people losing weight, So I made one more.

Then I made one more Role of Calories in Weight Loss. I got an even better response on YouTube and many more questions after that, I stopped making motivational videos and started making just weight loss videos to help people losing weight. My tips and plans are so easy and reality-based that people started losing weight with my plans. I started getting many appreciation comments and thanks also suggestions of new topics and money from YouTube monetization. I searched for research on the topic and made new videos every two days, and never looked back in just one year.

I have 161k subscribers on YouTube and approx. 175 videos on weight loss-related topics.

As much as I dived deep into fitness and weight loss study and making new videos covering various topics, for example, 1200 calories diet plan and intermittent fasting. People started contacting me on my Instagram for personal guidance and weight loss plans.

I did not have the qualifications to suggest people's diet plans but had the experience. So, I decided to upgrade myself, and I took admission in one of the most renowned and credible bodies in fitness and nutrition. Which is ISSA -

International Sports Sciences Association.

And started my certified personal trainer and sports nutritionist certification, which is currently undergoing.

So, this was my boring story of how I became a dietitian accidentally.

I believe some plans you make, and there are plans made for you if you work hard and have consistency to achieve something in life, no disease, no hurdle can stop you from becoming what you are meant to be.

In this book, I am sharing one of my diet plans in the next chapter, which helped many people lose fat and be fit. But if you have any disease, diabetes, blood pressure, or anything else, please follow this under your doctor or medical practitioner's supervision. Everybody acts differently, so taking a personal diet plan as per your need and general plans has vast differences in result.

CHAPTER 9
"MY FAT LOSS PLAN "

This is one of the most effective plans I have experienced and helped people losing weight and fat.

Disclaimer:

This plan is based on my experience and my clients' experiences. If you have any medical condition, please ask your doctor or medical practitioner first. I am not responsible for any kind of adverse health effects of this plan.

Breakfast

Breakfast is one of the most important meals of the day. This is when your body's clock restarts, and good healthy energy is required to spend the day efficiently. If you take an excellent high protein, high fiber breakfast, you feel fuller for longer and eat less in other meals.

I am a huge fan of Eggs, Oats, and Roti (Flat Bread). My plan is simple, inexpensive, and easy to make, so let's start.

WEEK 1: BREAKFAST

As you wake up, drink two glasses of room temperature water, slowly sip in 30 min and breakfast after 20 minutes.

Day 1:

Take-Two full hard Boil Eggs and 1 cup of Green Tea. Eggs are a good source of Protein and Fats 1 medium egg has approx.73 Calories.6.3 grams of protein. And 5.3 grams of fat. (Cholesterol Patients can take 1 Full Egg and 2 Whites)

Day 2:

Rolled Oats 3 Tbsp
Apple or Banana 1 Medium
Cinnamon Powder 1 Pinch
Chia Seeds 1 Tablespoon
Peanut Butter 1 Tablespoon (avoid peanut butter if you are allergic to peanuts; this can be life-threatening)

Cook 3 Tablespoon Rolled Oats in 1Cup Water or Skim Milk. After cooking, take the oats in a Bowl or Plate add one tablespoon peanut butter, one pinch of cinnamon, one tablespoon chia seeds, one apple or banana. Mix well and enjoy your breakfast with 1 cup of tea of your choice without sugar.

Day 3:

Take-Two full hard Boil Eggs and 1 cup Green Tea

Eggs are a good source of Protein and Fats 1 medium egg has approx.73 Calories.6.3 grams of protein. And 5.3 grams of fat.

(Cholesterol Patients can take 1 Full Egg and 2 Whites)

Day 4:

Barley Porridge 3 Tbsp

Strawberries or blueberries 5 to 8

Cinnamon powder 1 Pinch

Chia Seeds or Pumpkin Seeds 1 Tablespoon

Peanut Butter 1 Tablespoon (avoid peanut butter if you are allergic to peanut; this can be life-threatening)1

Cook 3 Tablespoon Barley Porridge in 1Cup Water or Skim Milk. After cooking, take the Porridge in a Bowl or Plate add one tablespoon peanut butter, one pinch of cinnamon, one tablespoon of seeds, berries. Mix well and enjoy your breakfast with 1 cup of tea of your choice without sugar.

Day 5:

Take-Two full hard Boil Eggs and 1 cup Green Tea

Eggs are a good source of Protein and Fats 1 medium egg has approx.73 Calories.6.3 grams of protein. And 5.3 grams of fat.

(Cholesterol Patients can take 1 Full Egg and 2 Whites).

Day 6:

Egg and Oats Omelet with 1 30 Gram Flat Bread of Whole wheat flour.

A Cup of Black Coffee

Day 7:

Quinoa or Oats Porridge 3 Tbsp

Dry Fruits 11 Almonds and 11 Cashew Nuts

Peanut Butter 1 Tablespoon

Pumpkin, Hemp, or Chia Seeds 1 Tbsp.

Cook the Porridge in 1 cup of water, add other ingredients and enjoy. Also, have two egg whites boiled and a cup of tea.

LUNCH

Drink a full glass of water right before a meal. It would help to eat less.

On Lunch Day 1 to 6, you will have vegetable and fruit salad mixing below mentioned vegetables only or vegetables and fruits of your choices along with 3 special things.

List of Vegetables

All green leafy vegetables, cucumber, radish, lettuce, rocket leaves, celery, salad leaves, onion, tomatoes, and vegetables of your choice avoid potatoes.

3 Special Things.

Along with vegetables, add chicken, White Chickpeas, or Red Kidney Beans 1 thing per day quantity approx. 100 grams.

(Note: Please cook Red Kidney Beans Properly for 10 or more minutes. Eating them undercooked or raw can be toxic).

Day 7

Eat Brown Rice 1 cup with Chicken Steams and Celery or Cucumber.

DINNER

Drink a full glass of water right before a meal. It would help to eat less. Finish your dinner 4 to 5 hours before sleep and no food or calories, only water.

Day 1:

Lentils Soup only No Rice No Bread. You can mix two lentils or legumes to enhance the quality of protein.

Day 2:

100 Gram Chicken Steamed, Grilled BBQ or Boiled with 1 Bran Bread Slice of Flatbread (Roti) 30 Gram Whole Wheat Flour.

Day 3:

Lentils Soup only No Rice No Bread. You can mix two lentils or legumes to enhance the quality of protein.

Day 4:

100 Gram grilled fish (Tuna or Salmon) with sautéed green vegetables.

Day 5:

Cabbage Soup with 2 Hard Boiled Eggs.

Day 6:

100 Gram Chicken Steamed, Grilled BBQ or Boiled with 1 Bran Bread Slice of Flatbread (Roti) 30 Gram Whole Wheat Flour.

Day 7:

Vegetable Salad with Chicken and chickpeas. 1 Bowl

WEEK 2: BREAKFAST

As you wake up, drink two glasses of room temperature water, slowly sip in 30 min and breakfast after 20 minutes.

Day 1:

2 egg whites scrambled with 2 whole grain bread slices.

Day 2:

Rolled Oats 3 Tbsp

Apple or Banana 1 Medium

Cinnamon Powder 1 Pinch

Chia Seeds 1 Tablespoon

Peanut Butter 1 Tablespoon (avoid peanut butter if you are allergic to peanut; this can be life-threatening)1

Cook 3 Tablespoon Rolled Oats in 1Cup Water or Skim Milk. After cooking, take the oats in a Bowl or Plate add 1 tablespoon peanut butter, 1 pinch of cinnamon, 1 tablespoon chia seeds, 1 apple or banana. Mix well and enjoy your breakfast with 1 cup of tea of your choice without sugar.

Day 3:

Egg and Oats Omelet with 1 Gram Flour Roti (Flatbread Bread home-cooked and 1 Green Tea.

Day 4:

Barley Porridge 3 Tbsp

Strawberries or blueberries 5 to 8

Cinnamon powder 1 Pinch

Chia Seeds or Pumpkin Seeds 1 Tablespoon

Peanut Butter 1 Tablespoon (avoid peanut butter if you are allergic to peanut; this can be life-threatening)1

Cook 3 Tablespoon Barley Porridge in 1Cup Water or Skim Milk. After cooking, take the Porridge in a Bowl or Plate add 1 tablespoon peanut butter, 1 pinch of cinnamon, 1 tablespoon seeds, berries. Mix well and enjoy your breakfast with 1 cup of tea of your choice without sugar.

Day 5:

Take-Two full hard Boil Eggs and 1 cup Green Tea

Eggs are a good source of Protein and Fats 1 medium egg has approx.73 Calories.6.3 grams of protein. And 5.3 grams of fat. (Cholesterol Patients can take 1 Full Egg and 2 Whites)

Day 6:

Two Egg Whites omelet with Veggies and low-fat cheese and 1 Flat Bread (Roti) Whole Wheat Flour 30 Gram

Day 7:

Quinoa or Oats Porridge 3 Tbsp

Dry Fruits 11 Almonds and 11 Cashew Nuts

Peanut Butter 1 Tablespoon

Pumpkin, Hemp, or Chia Seeds 1 Tbsp.

Cook the Porridge in 1 cup of water, add other ingredients and enjoy. Also, have two egg whites boiled and a cup of tea.

WEEK 2: LUNCH

Drink a full glass of water right before a meal. It would help to eat less.

On Lunch Day 1 to 6, you will have vegetable and fruit salad mixing below mentioned vegetables only or vegetables and fruits of your choices along with 3 special things.

List of Vegetables

All green leafy vegetables, cucumber, radish, lettuce, rocket leaves, celery, salad leaves, onion, tomatoes, and vegetables of your choice avoid potatoes.

3 Special Things.

Along with vegetables, add chicken, White Chickpeas, or Red Kidney Beans 1 thing per day quantity approx. 100 grams.

 (Note: Please cook Red Kidney Beans Properly for 10 or more minutes. Eating them undercooked or raw can be toxic)

Day 7

Eat Whole Grain Pasta with Chicken

WEEK 2: DINNER

Drink a full glass of water right before a meal. It would help to eat less. Finish your dinner 4 to 5 hours before sleep and no food or calories, only water.

Day 1:

1 Flat Bread (Roti) of Gram Flour Called Besan Ki Roti in Pakistan and India along with Mint Chutney and Yogurt.

Day 2:

100 Gram Chicken Steamed, Grilled BBQ or Boiled with 1 Bran Bread Slice of Flatbread (Roti) 30 Gram Whole Wheat Flour.

Day 3:

Cabbage Soup with 2 Hard Boiled Eggs.

Day 4:

100 Gram grilled fish (Tuna or Salmon) with sautéed green vegetables.

Day 5:

Pumpkin or Spinach cooked without Bread or Rice. You can add some low-fat cheese.

Day 6:

100 Gram Chicken Steamed, Grilled BBQ or Boiled with 1 Bran Bread Slice of Flatbread (Roti) 30 Gram Whole Wheat Flour.

Day 7:

Vegetable Salad with Chicken and chickpeas. 1 Bowl

 No snacks in between. Trust me, and you won't feel hungry for snacks. But if you do, just fruits allow.

No processed food, junk food, sugary drinks.

I shared two-week separate plans with you. You can try this for two months on an alternate basis; you can contact me on my Instagram for further plans.

@khawarLF

CHAPTER 9
"NOW WHO I AM "

 When we talk about Now, Now is the only real people see about you. Gone is gone, done is done. Winning or losing is entirely in your mind, and I am not a philosopher. I am just sharing what I feel and experience.

Work in your Now to make your Now Better. Whatever problem you have from relationship to financial to body weight. Stop taking the stress of things not in your control and start making small changes in your life for a significant change.

For example, Slowly and effectively eradicate white sugar and sugary drinks from your life.

Stop eating processed food. And start thinking positively about small little things to big problems.

I hope this book brings a good chance at least in a minute of your life; I will find efforts worth doing.

Have a good life ahead.